SEXUAL WELLNESS

NAVIGATING THE PATH TO HEALTHY SEXUALITY

KATE .P

Contents

CHAPTER ONE

INTRODUCTION

Welcome to "Sexual Wellness: Navigating the Path to Healthy Sexuality." This book seeks to offer a safe, enlightening, and inspiring environment for examining the complexity of sexual health and well-being in a world where conversations about sexuality are frequently taboo or surrounded by stigma.

More than simply physical health, sexual wellness includes all of our identities, relationships, and sexual experiences. It includes our capacity to make wise decisions regarding our bodies and relationships, as well as our mental, emotional, physical, and social well-being.

We will cover a wide range of subjects connected to sexual wellness in this book, including managing consent, communication, and healthy relationships, as well as understanding our own bodies and wants. We will examine the ways in which gender identity, sexual orientation, race, culture, and religion connect with sexuality to examine how these elements affect how we experience and understand sexuality.

On your road towards sexual wellness, you will find material based on evidence, useful advice, and firsthand accounts throughout these pages. This book will help you every step of the way, whether you're looking for advice on sexual health, exploring your own needs and boundaries, or trying to improve intimacy and connection in your relationships.

Above all, "Sexual Wellness" aims to advance a sex-positive, welcoming, and affirming perspective on sexuality—one that values consent and respect and celebrates variety and pleasure. We can dismantle obstacles, combat stigma, and enable people to proudly and confidently embrace their sexual identities and experiences by encouraging candid and open discussions about sexuality.

Together, let's set out on this road towards empowerment, self-awareness, and sexual wellbeing. I hope that this book may be useful to you as you travel the path to fulfilling relationships and healthy sexuality in your own life.

Comprehending Sexual Health

The physical, psychological, and social aspects of sexuality and sexual behavior are all included in the wide and complex concept of sexual health, which is a component of general well-being. It encompasses good things like enjoyment, closeness, and civil interactions in addition to the absence of illness or dysfunction. Several essential elements are involved in comprehending sexual health:

Physical Health: This includes the promotion of healthy reproductive systems, access to family planning and contraception, and the prevention and treatment of sexually transmitted diseases (STIs). It's crucial to get routine check-ups with medical professionals, engage in safe sexual behavior, and seek assistance when needed.

Emotional and Mental Health: Emotional and psychological components are also a part of sexual health. This include managing concerns like body image and self-esteem, comprehending and accepting one's gender identity and sexual orientation, and managing feelings associated with sexual experiences. Experts in mental health can provide assistance in addressing these problems.

Consent and Communication: The idea of consent, or the free decision to participate in sexual activity, is essential to maintaining good sexual health. Consent must be freely offered, unforced, and rescindable at any moment. In order to express needs, wants, and worries as well as negotiate sexual experiences and boundaries, one must be able to communicate effectively.

Healthy Relationships: Promoting courteous and satisfying relationships built on mutual understanding, communication, and trust is essential to sexual health. This entails identifying and resolving problems like abuse, coercion, and domestic violence. Constructive dispute resolution, empathy, and attentive listening are all necessary for developing strong relationships.

Sexual Pleasure: A crucial component of sexual health is acknowledging and giving priority to sexual pleasure. This entails examining one's own inclinations and preferences, learning about the anatomy and physiology of the sex, and looking for satisfying, consensual sexual encounters. Enhancing one's sexual enjoyment requires a combination of critical thinking, education, and self-awareness.

Cultural and Social Factors: Social attitudes, legislative frameworks pertaining to sexuality, and cultural norms all have an impact on sexual health. In order to promote inclusive and non-discriminatory sexual health practices and policies, it is imperative that varied viewpoints on sexuality, gender, and relationships be understood and respected.

Access to Resources and Services: It is essential for people to be able to make educated decisions about their sexual health that they have access to thorough sexual health education, information, and healthcare services. This covers the availability of contraception, STI screening and treatment, HIV prevention, counseling on sexual health, and support services for victims of sexual assault.

Recognizing the connections between the physical, emotional, social, and cultural elements that influence people's sexual experiences and well-being is essential to understanding sexual health. Encouraging sexual health necessitates all-encompassing strategies that take into account these different aspects and provide people the ability to make decisions that will improve their quality of life in general.

The Physiology and Anatomy of Sexual Function

In both males and females, the anatomy and physiology of sexual function entail a complex interplay of biological processes and structures. Here's a quick rundown:

Anatomy and physiology of male sexuality:

The external genitalia.

Penis: The penis is made up of three erectile tissue-filled cylindrical chambers. These chambers fill with blood when a person is sexually aroused, which makes the penis erect.

The testes are located in a pouch of skin called the scrotum. It aids in controlling the testicular temperature for optimum sperm production.

Internal Appendages:

Testes: The main male sex hormone, testosterone, and sperm are produced by the testes.

The epididymis is a coiled tube that stores and moves sperm on the rear of each testis.

Vas Deferens: During ejaculation, these ducts transport sperm from the epididymis to the ejaculatory duct.

Anatomical Mechanisms:

Erection: When sexually aroused, neurotransmitters are released into the penis, causing the smooth muscles to relax and allowing blood to enter the erectile chambers, resulting in an erection.

Ejaculation: Semen is propelled into the urethra and out of the penis by the repetitive contractions of pelvic floor muscles during an orgasm.

The anatomy and physiology of female sexuality

The external genitalia.

Clitoris: At the summit of the vulva is the extremely sensitive clitoris organ. It is the main source of erectile pleasure for women and contains erectile tissue.

Labia: The skin folds known as the labia majora and minora encircle the vaginal opening and shield the internal reproductive organs.

Internal Appendages:

Vagina: The entry to the reproductive tract is provided by the muscular canal known as the vagina. It also serves as a pathway for births and menstruation.

Uterus: During pregnancy, a fertilized egg implants and develops in the uterus, also known as the womb.

Ovaries: The ovaries secrete progesterone and estrogen, two female sex hormones, as well as eggs, or ova.

Anatomical Mechanisms:

Vasocongestion: Just like in men, women who are sexually aroused experience an increase in blood flow to the pelvic region, which enlarges the clitoris and vaginal tissues.

lubricant: Vaginal lubricant is released in response to arousal, reducing friction and improving comfort during sexual activity.

Orgasm: A period of extreme pleasure and tension release is accompanied by the rhythmic contraction of the pelvic floor muscles.

Numerous elements, including as hormonal balance, psychological state, relationship dynamics, and general health, can affect both male and female sexual performance. The significance of holistic approaches to sexual health and well-being is highlighted by the impact that dysfunction in any of these domains can have on sexual function and satisfaction.

Investigating Orientation and Sexual Identity

Understanding one's attraction, wants, and sense of self in relation to others is a crucial part of the deeply personal journey that is exploring one's sexual identity and orientation. Here are some important things to think about:

Comprehending Sexual Identity:

The word "sexual identity" describes how people view and identify their own sexuality in relation to their desires, activities, and sense of self.

It includes a variety of identities, such as asexual, bisexual, pansexual, gay, lesbian, and heterosexual. It's critical to understand that sexual identity is a spectrum concept that can change over time and be flexible.

In addition to sexual orientation, other facets of sexuality such as gender identity and romantic orientation can also be included in the concept of sexual identity.

Examining Sexual Attraction:

The gender or genders to which a person is attracted romantically or sexually are referred to as their sexual orientation. Typical categories consist of:

Attraction to people of the opposite gender is known as heterosexuality.

Attraction to people of the same gender is a sign of homosexuality.

Attraction to people of both genders is known as bisexuality.

Pansexuality is the attraction to people of any gender.

Asexual: Having little to no desire to mate.

Realizing that a person's sexual orientation is an intrinsic part of who they are rather than a choice is crucial. It can be found and accepted gradually via introspection and investigation.

Factors Affecting Orientation and Sexual Identity:

Biological Factors: A person's sexual orientation may be influenced by hormonal, neurological, and genetic factors.

Environmental and Social Factors: People's perceptions and expressions of their sexual identities can be influenced by their family, culture, religion, and society attitudes toward sexuality.

Personal Experience: An individual's perception of their sexual identity and orientation is greatly influenced by their own connections, experiences, and self-discovery.

Managing Identity and Disclosure:

Exploring and accepting one's sexual identity may be a difficult process for many people, frequently marked by societal stigma, fear, and bewilderment.

The act of disclosing to people one's gender identity or sexual orientation is referred to as coming out. This is a very personal choice that, depending on the circumstances, may happen gradually or all at once.

For people navigating their sexual identity and orientation, support from friends, family, and LGBTQ+ communities can be extremely helpful. Establishing secure and welcoming environments is crucial to enabling individuals to freely explore and express who they truly are.

Honoring Inclusivity and Diversity:

Respecting and validating the wide variety of sexual identities and orientations that exist in society is essential. Regardless of sexual orientation or identity, everyone deserves to be treated with respect, acceptance, and understanding.

In order to create a society that is more inclusive and affirming of all people, regardless of their sexual orientation or gender identity, it is imperative that advocates for LGBTQ+ rights take up the cause and confront prejudice and discrimination.

Investigating one's sexual orientation and identity is a very personal and continuous process. It's critical to approach it with candor, understanding, and a desire to develop both personally and as a group.

Boundaries, Communication, and Consent

Foundational components of healthy and respectful relationships, including sexual interactions, include consent, limits, and communication. It is essential to comprehend and give priority to these elements in order to foster mutual respect, safety, and autonomy. Below is an explanation of each:

Assent:

Definition of consent: The willing, enthusiastic, and shared decision to partake in a particular sexual activity is known as consent. It must be offered voluntarily, free from manipulation or coercion, and it is always withdrawable.

Important Ideas:

Explicitness: Consent must be expressed in a way that leaves no room for doubt, either by words or deeds.

Capacity: In order to grant permission, both participants must be of legal age, mentally sound, and free from any drugs or alcohol that could affect their judgment.

Continuity: Obtaining and confirming consent is a continual process that needs to happen during all sexual activity. Permission for one kind of behavior does not imply permission for another.

Communication: Gaining and keeping consent depend on effective communication. Asking for consent, paying attention to cues both spoken and unspoken, and honoring any reluctance or denial are all part of this.

Limitations:

Definition: Boundaries are individual restrictions and choices pertaining to encounters that are sexual, emotional, and physical. They specify what each partner can feel at ease and what is appropriate in a relationship.

Different Boundaries:

Physical Boundaries: These include preferences for physical contact and intimacy, such as kissing, touching, or engaging in sexual activities.

CHAPTER TWO

Emotional Boundaries: These include sharing emotions or talking about personal experiences. They also have to do with feelings, vulnerability, and emotional intimacy.

Social Boundaries: These include choices about social relationships, private areas, and solitude, including spending time alone or with people.

Communication and Respect: Respecting others' boundaries entails being aware of their limitations, being explicit about one's own, and reacting to others' boundaries with empathy. It's critical to understand that boundaries can differ from person to person and might change over time.

Interaction:

Open and Sincere Communication: It takes effective communication to convey needs, wants, and concerns and to comprehend those of a partner. This covers speaking, listening intently, and showing empathy.

Active Consent: When boundaries, wants, and wishes are discussed honestly, it creates an environment where both parties feel free to voice their opinions and bargain for what they need.

Handling Tough Talks: It's critical to establish a secure and accepting environment for talking about touchy subjects like sexual preferences, painful memories, or boundary concerns. Patience, sensitivity, and mutual respect are essential for negotiating these discussions.

People can develop happy, healthy relationships based on mutual respect, trust, and understanding by emphasizing consent, honoring boundaries, and encouraging open communication. Establishing a culture of respect and dignity in all interactions, including sexual ones, and fostering emotional well-being all depend on these behaviors.

Preventative health measures and safe sexual practices

In order to lower the risk of STIs and unwanted pregnancies, safe sex practices and preventative healthcare measures are essential. The following are some essential behaviors:

Use of Condoms:

HIV risk can be considerably decreased by consistently and properly using condoms during oral, anal, and vaginal sex.

For each sexual act, apply a fresh condom made of latex or polyurethane.

Water-based lubricants can lessen friction and the likelihood that a condom will break.

Frequent Testing for STIs:

Get STI testing done on a regular basis, particularly if you participate in high-risk sexual conduct or have several sexual partners.

Among the common sexually transmitted infections (STIs) include gonorrhea, syphilis, HIV, herpes, and human papillomavirus (HPV).

In order to control any potential health consequences and stop the spread of STIs, early testing and treatment are crucial.

Speaking with Partners:

Before having sex, talk to your partner about your sexual health and STI status.

Ask partners about their STI status and be forthright and honest about your own.

Transparency and mutual disclosure can support each partner's decision-making and precaution-taking.

Restricting Sexual Partners:

To lower your chance of contracting STIs, cut down on the number of sexual partners you have.

A mutually faithful partner in a monogamous relationship can reduce the incidence of sexually transmitted infections.

HIV Prevention using PrEP and PEP:

For those who are at high risk of HIV exposure, pre-exposure prophylaxis (PrEP) entails taking a daily medicine (such as Truvada or Descovy) to lower the chance of HIV transmission.

Antiretroviral therapy must be taken within 72 hours of possible HIV contact as part of post-exposure prophylaxis (PEP) to avoid infection.

Additional preventative interventions, such as PrEP and PEP, are recommended for those who are at a higher risk of HIV transmission, such as those who have HIV-positive partners or participate in high-risk sexual conduct.

Shots to Prevent STDs:

There are vaccines available to prevent hepatitis B and HPV, among other STIs.

It is advised that both men and women get the HPV vaccine in order to protect against genital warts and malignancies linked to HPV.

Healthcare professionals and those who are sexually active are among the groups of people who should get vaccinated against hepatitis B.

Frequent examinations for reproductive and gynecological health:

Regular gynecological exams, which include Pap smears and STI testing, are recommended for women.

To make well-informed decisions regarding family planning and contraception, talk to healthcare professionals about available contraceptive methods and issues related to reproductive health.

Steer clear of risky behaviors:

Steer clear of sharing needles or other drug paraphernalia as this raises the possibility of contracting hepatitis and HIV, two bloodborne illnesses.

Even while under the influence of drugs or alcohol, use safer sexual practices since impairment might result in unsafe sexual activity.

People can protect themselves and their partners against STIs and unwanted pregnancies by implementing these safe sex practices and preventive health measures into their sexual activity, thereby boosting overall sexual health and well-being.

Pleasure and satisfaction from sex

Physical, emotional, and relational factors, among others, all have an impact on sexual pleasure and satisfaction, which are crucial components of overall well-being. Here are some important things to think about:

Comprehending Eroticism:

The physical and emotional experiences that accompany sexual activity and lead to emotions of arousal, satisfaction, and enjoyment are referred to as sexual pleasure.

A wide range of feelings, such as arousal, desire, orgasm, intimacy, and emotional ties with a partner, may be included.

Because it is subjective, sexual enjoyment varies widely across people and is impacted by a variety of things, including experiences, wants, and personal preferences.

Variables Affecting Sexual Pleasure:

Physical Factors: Hormonal balance, sexual anatomy, general health, and other physical factors can all have an impact on how pleasurable sexual activity is. Pleasure can be enhanced by knowledge of one's own body and sexual responses.

Emotional Factors: Feelings of closeness, trust, and emotional intimacy with a partner are important components of sexual pleasure. Sexual fulfillment can be improved by feeling understood, safe, and valued.

Relational Factors: Mutual awareness of boundaries and desires, communication with a partner, and the quality of the relationship all play a role in promoting sexual enjoyment.

Enhancing emotional closeness and trust might increase sexual enjoyment.

Psychological variables: Sexual enjoyment can be impacted by psychological variables like stress, anxiety, body image problems, and traumatic events. Taking care of underlying psychological issues might enhance one's sexual health.

Exploration and Variety: Experimenting with various imaginations, techniques, and sexual activities can improve the pleasure and satisfaction of sex. Experimentation and discovery can be aided by having open discussion about interests and wants with a partner.

Self-Exploration: Sexual happiness and confidence can be enhanced by self-pleasure (masturbation) and self-exploration, which help one understand their own desires, preferences, and boundaries.

Improving Eroticism and Sexual Pleasure:

Enhancing sexual enjoyment requires open and honest conversation with a partner regarding preferences, boundaries, and aspirations. Having a conversation about likes, dislikes, and dreams can result in more satisfying sex.

Extended foreplay, which entails kissing, caressing, and sensuous touch, can raise desire and improve sexual enjoyment for both parties.

variation and Novelty: Adding variation and novelty to sexual activities, such experimenting with different poses, settings, or sensual games, helps maintain the excitement and fulfillment of sexual encounters.

Emotional Connection: You can increase your level of sexual satisfaction and have a more satisfying relationship outside of the bedroom by developing emotional intimacy and connection with your partner.

Self-Care: Making self-care, relaxation, and stress reduction a priority can boost libido and general well-being.

All things considered, a mix of relational, emotional, and physical components contribute to sexual pleasure and satisfaction. Individuals and couples can nurture rewarding and happy sexual encounters that enhance general happiness and well-being by being aware of and giving priority to these factors.

Close Relationships and Healthy Sexual Development

As they offer a setting for expressing desires, feeling close, and forming emotional bonds, intimate relationships are important in forming sexual well-being. This is how having close relationships affects one's sexual health:

Emotional Bonding and Confidence:

Emotional closeness, trust, and respect are the foundations of intimate partnerships. A sense of safety and comfort is fostered when one feels emotionally connected and comfortable with a partner, and this is crucial for sexual well-being.

A person can have more emotional and sexual intimacy with their partner when they feel comfortable being open and vulnerable with them.

Talking and Listening:

Good communication is essential to both sexual and intimate relationship wellness. Communicating openly with a partner about needs, expectations, and worries fosters satisfaction and understanding on both sides.

Efficient communication facilitates couples' needs expression, exploration of novel sexual experiences, and resolution of any obstacles or problems that may come up.

Respect for one another and consent:

Intimate relationships require respect for each other's individuality, limits, and choices in order to support healthy sexual behavior. Prioritizing mutual consent is important, and both partners should make sure that any sexual action is both desired and consensual.

Respecting one another's limits and inclinations creates a safe and trusting atmosphere that improves emotional and sexual fulfillment.

Mutual Closeness and Bonding:

Opportunities for closeness and shared experiences are presented by intimate relationships, both inside and outside of the bedroom. Interactions that foster emotional intimacy like spending time together, showing affection, and expressing gratitude fortify the relationship between partners and improve sexual health.

Hugging, kissing, and other forms of physical love strengthen emotional ties and foster a sense of intimacy and closeness.

Sexual Discovery and Satisfaction:

There is room for sexual experimentation, exploration, and fulfillment in intimate partnerships. In a secure and encouraging setting, partners can explore each other's imaginations, preferences, and desires, which improves sexual satisfaction and wellbeing.

A more meaningful sexual relationship results from couples prioritizing mutual pleasure and fulfillment through awareness of each other's wants and preferences.

Flexibility and Expansion:

Over time, intimate partnerships change, necessitating growth and adaptation from both parties. Together, navigating shifts in interests, preferences, and life circumstances improves long-term sexual well-being and deepens the link between lovers.

Resilience and increased sexual satisfaction in relationships are fostered by embracing openness to change, being honest about changing needs, and encouraging each other's development.

Overall, because they offer chances for emotional connection, communication, respect for one another, and sexual fulfillment, intimate relationships are essential for fostering sexual well-being. Couples that prioritize these areas of their relationship can develop a pleasant and rewarding sexual connection, which enhances happiness and well-being in general.

Healthy Sexual Behavior Throughout Life

A person's sexual health is a crucial component of their overall wellbeing, which changes throughout the course of their life due to a variety of biological, psychological, social, and cultural factors. Considerations for sexual health at various life phases are as follows:

Early Life and Teenage Years:

Sexual health education for children starts with age-appropriate conversations about personal safety, limits, and body awareness.

Physical changes, the investigation of one's sexual identity and orientation, and the emergence of sexual desire are all hallmarks of adolescence, a crucial time for sexual development.

Adolescents can receive correct information on puberty, contraception, STIs, consent, and healthy relationships via comprehensive sexual health education programs.

Early Adulthood:

Exploring romantic and sexual relationships, developing a sexual identity, and deciding on one's own sexual behavior are characteristics of young adulthood.

During this phase, safe sexual practices such as using condoms and avoiding STIs are crucial for preventing STIs and unwanted pregnancies.

Promoting sexual well-being requires having access to sexual health services, such as STI testing, reproductive health counseling, and contraception.

Growing Up:

Many sexual experiences, such as dating, committed partnerships, and motherhood, occur during adulthood.

STI testing on a regular basis, safe sex practices, and seeking medical assistance for concerns related to sexual health are all part of maintaining sexual health.

Sexual satisfaction and well-being can be impacted by relationship dynamics, stress, and life changes; this emphasizes the significance of communication and closeness in close relationships.

Beyond Midlife:

Although sexual activity may alter with age due to factors including menopause, health issues, and relationship dynamics, sexual health is still important in midlife and beyond.

Medical interventions or modifications in sexual habits may be necessary to address age-related changes in sexual function, such as erectile dysfunction or vaginal dryness.

In older life, maintaining emotional closeness and connection with a spouse might improve well-being and sexual satisfaction.

Senior Citizens:

Even though older persons may engage in less sexual activity, sexual health is still vital.

Intimacy problems, sexual dysfunction, and STI transmission are examples of sexual health difficulties that may call for specialist care and assistance catered to the requirements of older persons.

Encouraging interpersonal relationships, physical exercise, and general well-being can all support senior sexual health and enjoyment.

Promoting sexual health across the life span requires all-encompassing strategies that take into account the relational, emotional, social, and physical facets of sexuality. This entails having access to reliable sexual health information, receiving supportive medical care, and fostering an environment that values the variety of sexual identities and experiences. Through lifelong prioritization of sexual health, people can improve their general health and quality of life.

In the Digital Age, Sexual Health

The digital age has brought about a number of changes to the way people communicate with one another, access information, and engage in sexual activity, which has both benefits and concerns for sexual health. The impact of the digital era on sexual health is as follows:

Information Availability:

A plethora of information about sexual health is easily accessible online, including links to resources about STIs, contraception, sexual pleasure, and relationship guidance.

Social media, websites, and forums are examples of online platforms that provide people with the ability to seek information anonymously, hence lowering stigma and impediments to using services related to sexual health.

Sexual Behavior Online:

Opportunities for casual sex and hookups have expanded as a result of the way that dating apps and other media platforms have changed how individuals meet, flirt, and enter into relationships.

CHAPTER THREE

If safe sex practices are not followed, engaging in sexual activity online may raise the risk of STIs and unwanted pregnancies. This emphasizes the significance of education and access to sexual health care.

Sexual Advocacy and Education:

Digital platforms offer avenues for sexual health advocacy and education, such as social media outreach, webinars, and online campaigns.

Advocacy initiatives have the potential to advance inclusive sexual health education, confront stigma and prejudice, and increase public knowledge of reproductive justice and sexual rights.

Pornography on the Internet:

Online pornography has been widely accessible, which has affected expectations, attitudes, and actions around sexuality, especially among youth.

Concerns over pornography's possible detrimental impacts on relationships and sexual health are raised by the way it can affect how people perceive their bodies, their sexuality, and their consent.

Online healthcare and telemedicine:

Convenient access to sexual health treatments, such as virtual consultations with healthcare specialists, prescription renewals for contraception, and home delivery of STI testing kits, is made possible by telemedicine and online healthcare services.

Accessing sexual health treatments can be facilitated by online healthcare, which can help with issues like privacy and confidentiality, mobility, and geographic location.

Safety of Digital Dating:

Particularly for marginalized populations like LGBTQ+ persons and people of color, digital networks pose hazards of sexual harassment, coercion, and exploitation.

Campaigns for education and awareness, which include advice on establishing limits, confirming identities, and seeing indications of manipulation or abuse online, can help advance digital dating safety.

Security and Privacy Issues:

Online privacy and security dangers associated with sharing intimate or sexual content include the possibility of data breaches, revenge porn, and online abuse.

In order to address privacy and security concerns about digital platforms and online sexual conduct, advocacy work and legal protections are required.

In conclusion, the digital era has transformed how people approach sexual health by providing unparalleled access to data, tools, and medical care. But it also brings with it difficulties like internet threats, false information, and moral dilemmas. In the digital age, people can encourage positive results for sexual health by utilizing technology responsibly and supporting inclusive sexual health practices.

Since both components of well-being influence and support one another, sexual health and mental health are strongly related. The following is the relationship between mental health and sexual health:

Happy Sexual Encounters and Mental Well-Being:

Pleasure, intimacy, and mutual satisfaction are hallmarks of positive sexual experiences, which can be good to mental health.

Stress, worry, and depression can be lessened by engaging in sexual activity because it releases endorphins and other neurotransmitters that enhance sensations of pleasure and relaxation.

Consensual and mutually rewarding relationships that allow for healthy sexual expression promote emotional intimacy, connection, and a sense of belonging all of which are critical for mental health in general.

Mental Health and Sexual Dysfunction:

Sexual dysfunction, including low libido or erectile dysfunction, can cause distress and have a detrimental effect on mental health.

People who are having problems with their sexuality may feel nervous, angry, or inadequate, which can cause melancholy, low self-esteem, or difficulty in relationships.

It is crucial to treat underlying psychological difficulties, such as relationship problems, stress, or trauma, in order to manage sexual dysfunction and advance mental health.

Mental Health and Sexual Trauma:

Experiences of sexual trauma, such as abuse, harassment, or assault, can have a significant and enduring impact on one's mental state.

Sexual trauma survivors may exhibit signs of anxiety, sadness, or post-traumatic stress disorder (PTSD), among other mental health issues.

It is imperative that survivors have access to trauma-informed care, counseling, and support services in order to address the psychological effects of sexual trauma and promote healing.

LGBTQ+ people may experience particular difficulties that have an influence on their mental health and are related to their gender identity and sexual orientation.

Disparities in mental health among LGBTQ+ groups and minority stress can be caused by discrimination, stigma, and a lack of social support.

Promoting mental well-being within these communities requires fostering environments that are affirming and inclusive, offering healthcare that is culturally sensitive, and speaking out for the rights of LGBTQ+ people.

Education on Sexual Health and Mental Health:

By encouraging a sense of agency, self-esteem, and resilience, comprehensive sexual health education that supports positive attitudes, healthy relationships, and informed decision-making can boost mental well-being.

People may make educated decisions and navigate sexual experiences safely and confidently if they have access to correct information on consent, sexual health, and healthy relationships.

Handling Concerns About Co-occurring Sexual and Mental Health:

When mental health and sexual health services are combined, it can help those with co-occurring disorders achieve better results.

Approaches to collaborative care that attend to the requirements of both sexual and mental health can promote recovery and overall well-being and offer comprehensive support.

both mental and sexual health are entwined facets of total well-being that both support and influence one another. Individuals and communities can improve both sexual and mental well-being through establishing inclusive environments, addressing sexual dysfunction and trauma, encouraging good sexual experiences, and integrating sexual health and mental health care.

Reproductive rights and sexual health

Reproductive rights and sexual health are related ideas that cover people's autonomy, well-being, and dignity in regard to their sexual and reproductive life. This is how they come together:

Sexual well-being and the right to procreate:

The physical, emotional, mental, and social facets of sexuality and sexual activity are all included in sexual health. Access to complete sexual education, contraception, STI prevention and treatment, enjoyment of sexual activities, and reproductive health services are all included.

The term "reproductive rights" refers to people's ability to make choices regarding their reproductive lives, such as whether or not to have children, how many and how soon to have them, having access to reproductive health services, and being able to make educated decisions about abortion and contraception.

Obtaining Services for Sexual and Reproductive Health:

Promoting sexual health and reproductive rights requires ensuring access to services related to these topics. This covers getting access to safe and authorized abortion, prenatal care, STI testing and treatment, and maternal health services.

Accessibility obstacles can make it more difficult for people to exercise their freedom to sexual orientation and reproduction and to obtain necessary medical care. These obstacles can include lack of funds, stigma, governmental regulations, and restricted service availability.

All-inclusive Sexual Education

One essential element of sexual health and reproductive rights is comprehensive sexual education. It gives people accurate, age-appropriate knowledge about consent, healthy relationships, STIs, anatomy, puberty, contraception, and reproductive rights.

Comprehensive sexual education encourages tolerance for variety and inclusivity, gives people the power to make educated decisions about their sexual and reproductive health, and aids in the reduction of STIs and unwanted pregnancies.

Contraception and Family Planning:

It is essential for people to have access to family planning services and contraception in order to exercise their right to self-determination on when and whether to have children.

Barrier techniques, hormonal techniques, long-acting reversible contraceptives (LARCs), and emergency contraception should all be accessible and available.

By enabling people to plan and space out their pregnancies, contraception lowers the likelihood of unwanted pregnancies and abortions while also enhancing the health of mothers and children.

Rights Regarding Abortion:

One essential element of sexual health care and reproductive rights is having access to safe and legal abortion. Legal limits on abortion have the potential to increase maternal mortality, promote unsafe abortion procedures, and violate people's rights to bodily integrity and autonomy.

CHAPTER FOUR

Safe and legal access to abortion services preserves people's reproductive rights and dignity while also protecting their health and saving lives.

Dealing with Discrimination and Stigma:

Access to sexual and reproductive health care can be hampered by stigma and prejudice, which can also be detrimental to people's rights and general wellbeing.

Improving sexual health and reproductive rights for all people requires fostering stigma-free environments, opposing discriminatory laws and policies, and standing out for the rights of disadvantaged and underprivileged groups.

To sum up, reproductive rights and sexual health are essential components of peoples' autonomy, dignity, and well-being. Promoting sexual and reproductive rights and achieving international public health objectives depend on ensuring access to comprehensive sexual education, contraception, STI prevention and treatment, safe and legal abortion, and reproductive health care.

Sexual Trauma and Recovery

Any unwanted or non-consensual sexual experience that harms a person physically, emotionally, or psychologically is referred to as sexual trauma. The process of recovering from sexual trauma is unique to each person and might entail a variety of tactics and treatments. In order to comprehend sexual trauma and encourage healing, keep the following points in mind:

Acknowledging the Effects of Sexual Trauma

Survivors of sexual trauma may experience intense and long-lasting impacts, such as emotions of betrayal, fear, shame, and guilt.

A wide range of psychological and physiological symptoms, including as anxiety, despair, PTSD, dissociation, nightmares, flashbacks, and trouble trusting people, can affect survivors.

It's critical to understand that every trauma survivor's experience is distinct and that recovery is a highly personalized process.

Establishing a Secure and Helpful Environment

In order for survivors to feel acknowledged, believed, and empowered to ask for assistance and support, it is imperative to provide a safe and supportive environment.

Healing and recovery can be aided by giving survivors access to private, judgment-free support services like advocacy, counseling, and crisis intervention.

Looking for Expert Assistance:

For survivors of sexual trauma, expert assistance from therapists, counselors, or psychologists who specialize in trauma-informed treatment can be helpful in their processing and recovery.

Treatment approaches including dialectical behavior therapy (DBT), eye movement desensitization and reprocessing (EMDR), trauma-focused therapy, cognitive-behavioral therapy (CBT), and DBT may be beneficial in addressing symptoms associated with trauma and fostering healing.

Taking Part in Self-Care Activities:

Self-care techniques can aid in the healing process and assist survivors in overcoming the impacts of trauma. This could involve exercises, journaling, yoga, mindfulness meditation, creative expression, physical activity, and time spent in nature.

Resilience and general well-being can also be supported by placing a high priority on physical health, diet, sleep, and relaxation.

Developing Cordial Connections:

Developing connections of trust with family, friends, or support groups can help survivors feel understood, validated, and empathetic.

Developing relationships with people who have gone through comparable experiences helps lessen feelings of loneliness and foster a sense of belonging.

Examining Therapeutic Approaches:

Investigating complementary and alternative therapy techniques including art therapy, music therapy, acupuncture, massage therapy, and mindfulness-based practices might aid in healing.

various tactics or activities may be useful to various survivors in their recovery process, therefore it's important to experiment and figure out what suits each survivor's requirements and preferences.

Fighting for Accountability and Justice:

A crucial step in the healing process for survivors of sexual assault is holding those responsible for the abuse accountable and seeking justice. This could be filing a police report, taking legal action, or taking part in campaigns to oppose oppressive and violent systems and increase public awareness.

Recovering from sexual trauma is a difficult and non-linear process that calls for tolerance, understanding, and assistance. Communities may encourage healing and provide survivors the tools they need to take back control of their lives and futures by placing a high priority on their autonomy, dignity, and well-being and by giving them access to a wide range of resources and services.

Diversity and Inclusion in Sexuality

Beyond heterosexuality and cisgender identities, a vast array of sexual orientations, gender identities, and expressions are included in sexual diversity and inclusion. Establishing settings that accept, value, and affirm people of various sexual orientations and gender identities is a key component in promoting sexual diversity and inclusion. Here's how to promote inclusivity and variety in sexuality:

Recognizing Gender Identity and Sexual Orientation:

A person's emotional, romantic, or sexual attraction to another person is referred to as their sexual orientation. Heterosexual, homosexual (gay or lesbian), bisexual, pansexual, asexual, and other sexual orientations are common.

A person's internal perception of their gender, which may or may not correspond with the sex they were assigned at birth, is referred to as their gender identity. Male, female, non-binary, genderqueer, genderfluid, and other identities are examples of gender identities.

Increasing Knowledge and Informed Consciousness:

Promoting comprehension and acceptance of sexual diversity and inclusiveness requires education and awareness.

Information on sexual orientation, gender identity, consent, healthy relationships, and LGBTQ+ rights should all be covered in comprehensive sexual health education.

Teachers, medical professionals, employers, and community leaders can all benefit from training in order to better accept and affirm people with a variety of sexual orientations and gender identities.

Building Inclusive Environments:

Establishing situations where people feel comfortable, respected, and valued regardless of their gender identity or sexual orientation is a key component of creating inclusive spaces.

This could entail putting non-discrimination rules into place, speaking inclusively, and offering facilities that are gender-neutral.

Using outward symbols, like pride flags or LGBTQ+ resource centers, to publicly affirm LGBTQ+ identities can also contribute to a feeling of acceptance and belonging.

Taking On Discrimination and Stigma:

It is imperative to confront stigma and discrimination directed towards LGBTQ+ individuals in order to advance sexual diversity and inclusivity.

This could entail dispelling myths, fighting for the rights of LGBTQ+ people, and speaking out against laws and policies that discriminate.

Helping LGBTQ+ people who encounter harassment or discrimination can build resilience and legitimize their experiences.

Encouragement of LGBTQ+ Health and Welfare:

Giving LGBTQ+ people access to affirming healthcare services that cater to their particular needs and concerns is essential to promoting their health and well-being.

Training on LGBTQ+ health inequalities, cultural competency, and inclusive practices should be provided to healthcare providers.

LGBTQ+ people may benefit from mental health services, such as counseling and support groups, to help them deal with the stress of being a minority and the difficulties of coming out.

Promoting the Rights of LGBTQ+ People:

In order to advocate for LGBTQ+ rights, one must support legislative and policy measures that advance equality, anti-discrimination, and LGBTQ+ rights.

This could entail supporting legislation against discrimination, transgender rights, marriage equality, and LGBTQ+ people's access to healthcare.

It helps dispel misconceptions and advance acceptance when LGBTQ+ people and communities are celebrated for their diversity and visibility.

Pride celebrations, LGBTQ+ history months, and other festivities offer chances to commemorate accomplishments, increase awareness, and foster a sense of community.

In conclusion, deliberate efforts to advance knowledge, acceptance, and affirmation of people of all sexual orientations and gender identities are necessary to develop sexual diversity and inclusion. Communities may build an equal and welcoming society for all by fostering inclusive environments, combating stigma and prejudice, promoting LGBTQ+ rights, fostering health and well-being, and appreciating variety.

Honoring Sexual Expression and Diversity

Recognizing and respecting the vast array of sexual orientations, gender identities, and expressions that exist in society is a necessary part of celebrating sexual diversity and expression. It's about encouraging acceptance, respect, and inclusion for every person and acknowledging that every person's sexual orientation and gender identity are distinct and legitimate. Here are some ideas for honoring the variety and expression of sexuality:

Affirmation and Visibility:

Make sure that a variety of gender identities and sexual orientations are honored and portrayed in literature, art, media, and cultural events.

Emphasize the accomplishments and contributions made by LGBTQ+ people and communities in the arts, politics, science, history, and other sectors.

By giving LGBTQ+ creators, artists, and activists a platform and telling their story, you can support them.

Take part in festivals, parades, and pride events honoring LGBTQ+ identities, accomplishments, and history.

Participating in pride events, volunteering, or donating to LGBTQ+ organizations are ways to show your support for LGBTQ+ communities.

CHAPTER FIVE

Take use of pride celebrations to promote equality, educate the public about LGBTQ+ rights, and strengthen ties within the community.

Knowledge and Consciousness:

Through workshops, trainings, and educational materials, educate yourself and others about topics related to gender identity, sexual orientation, and LGBTQ+ community.

Organize talks or activities that advance empathy, tolerance, and allyship for LGBTQ+ people and communities.

In order to raise awareness and lessen stigma, provide LGBTQ+ inclusive sexual health education in community settings, colleges, and schools.

Conducive Conditions:

Establish welcoming environments where people of all gender identities and sexual orientations feel appreciated, safe, and respected.

Put nondiscrimination rules into place and train volunteers and employees on LGBTQ+ inclusiveness and cultural sensitivity.

Provide facilities and restrooms that are gender-neutral to accommodate people with varying gender identities.

Verifying Symbols and Words:

Speak in a way that is inclusive of people of different gender identities and sexual orientations, affirming and respecting them.

To show support and acceptance, display LGBTQ+ symbols like pride flags and inclusive signage.

Respect people's self-identification and refrain from making assumptions about their gender identity or sexual orientation.

Building Community and Solidarity:

Create systems of support and community networks that offer LGBTQ+ people and their supporters advocacy, resources, and social ties.

Encourage allyship and solidarity amongst various communities to enhance communication, cooperation, and group effort.

Speak out against acts of violence, harassment, and discrimination directed towards LGBTQ+ people, and back initiatives aimed at advancing justice and equality for all.

Honoring Uniqueness and Expression of Self:

Urge people to freely and truthfully disclose their gender identity and sexual orientation.

Honor the variety of gender identities, sexual orientations, and expressions that exist within your own community and stand up for people's freedom to choose how they want to express themselves.

Accept and appreciate the sexuality that you choose to express yourself, and help others to do the same.

It is important to embrace the range and complexity of gender identity and human sexuality in order to celebrate sexual diversity and expression. Regardless of one's gender identity or sexual orientation, we can all live in a more supportive and affirming society if we work to increase acceptance, visibility, and inclusion.

Thoughts on the Path to Sexual Wellness

Exploration, self-discovery, and personal development are all part of the complex and incredibly personal process that is the path to sexual wellbeing. Some thoughts on this voyage are as follows:

Self-Awareness and Sincerity:

Self-acceptance and embracing one's distinct sexual identity, wants, and boundaries are the first steps toward sexual wellbeing.

A rewarding and genuine sexual encounter begins with accepting and celebrating who you are, without guilt or condemnation.

Investigating and Being Curious:

People who are sexually healthy are free to explore and learn about their own bodies, wants, and preferences. It's a journey of inquiry and discovery.

Enhancing sexual pleasure and deepening closeness with others and oneself can be achieved through being receptive to new experiences, fantasies, and sensations.

Interaction and Communication:

Sexual wellbeing requires effective communication, both with one's sexual partners and with oneself.

A safe and encouraging environment for sexual exploration and expression is created when needs, boundaries, and wants are communicated.

This promotes closeness, mutual understanding, and respect.

Being Present and Mindful:

Enhancing pleasure and strengthening bonds during intercourse can be achieved through practicing mindfulness and presence.

People who are totally present in the moment are able to tune into their own feelings and reactions, which fosters a more profound sense of closeness and fulfillment.

Limitations and Assent:

Sexual wellbeing depends on consenting to sexual activity and respecting one's own boundaries.

Setting consent as a top priority guarantees that all parties have respectful, empowered, and consenting sexual interactions.

Emotional Health:

Emotional well-being and sexual wellbeing go hand in hand because emotional closeness and connection increase sexual satisfaction.

A stronger sense of fulfillment and connection is fostered in relationships through fostering emotional intimacy, trust, and vulnerability.

Self-Management and Wellbeing Techniques:

Making wellbeing and self-care a priority promotes general sexual well-being.

Physical and mental well-being are enhanced by practicing mindfulness, exercise, relaxation techniques, and getting enough sleep. These factors all have a good impact on sexual wellness.

Ongoing Development and Education:

The path to sexual wellbeing is one of ongoing learning, development, and evolution.

People can enhance their understanding of sexuality and strengthen their bonds with others and themselves by keeping an open mind to new experiences, viewpoints, and discoveries.

Self-compassion and Resilience:

Developing self-compassion and resilience are crucial components of sexual wellness.

People may traverse the complexity of sexuality with more comfort and self-compassion when they acknowledge and learn from their struggles, setbacks, and weaknesses.

Support and Community:

Getting help from dependable friends, lovers, or experts can be very helpful when pursuing sexual wellness.

Making connections with encouraging groups, whether virtual or real-world, offers affirmation, inspiration, and a feeling of inclusion.

All things considered, the path to sexual wellbeing is a highly intimate and life-changing one that entails self-awareness, development, and connection. Through embracing communication, self-care, authenticity, and ongoing education, people can develop a positive and powerful relationship with their sexuality, which enhances their general happiness and well-being.

summary

To sum up, sexual health is an essential component of total well-being, which includes relational, emotional, and physical aspects. Anatomy and physiology, sexual identity and orientation, consent and communication, safe sex practices, sexual pleasure and satisfaction, intimate relationships, sexual diversity and inclusion, sexual trauma and healing, and the celebration of sexual diversity and expression are just a few of the topics we've covered throughout this exploration of various aspects of sexual health.

As we've discovered, sexual health includes more than just the absence of illness or dysfunction it also includes good qualities like fulfillment, pleasure, and intimacy. It calls for honest communication, respect for one another's identities, and acceptance of differences in experiences. In order to promote sexual health, one must establish surroundings that are encouraging, confront stigma and prejudice, stand up for rights and access to care, and encourage personal agency and empowerment.

We can build a more welcoming, equal, and affirming society where everyone may lead joyful sexual lives by encouraging sexual health and well-being at all ages and among a variety of demographics. It's critical to carry on the conversation, push for reform, and back programs that advance everyone's rights, dignity, and sexual health. Working together, we can create a future in which sexual health is recognized as essential to human flourishing and is treated with respect and priority.

THE END